Chakras for Beginners

The Complete Guide to Balance your Chakras. Learn How to Use Your Inner Energy to Heal Your Mind and Body, and Achieve All Your Goals.

Sunny Heal

Table of Contents

Introduction

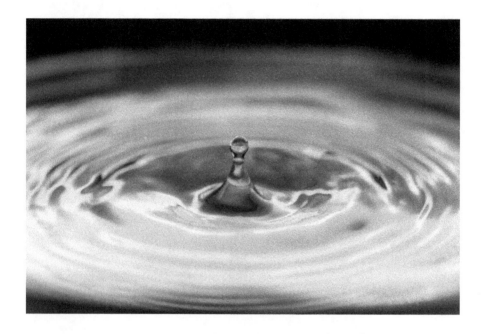

Dear reader, thank you for choosing *Chakras for Beginners.*
The following chapters will bring you into the discuss on the
concept of chakras and the role they have played in human
history over the course of several millennia. By the end of this
reading, you will know about chakras and their role in every
person's life. You will learn how chakras work and why
everyone should take care of their chakras.

The concept of chakras is an ancient one, filled with mystery as it evolves over time to become one of the most popular energetic models to explain how humans interact with the unseen world around us. The ideas that we live in our physical world, as well as a more subtle, energetic or spiritual world, are key to these philosophies and concepts.

The acceptance of chakras is the step that needs to be taken to cross this threshold and open many paths for other concepts to make their way to the west.

In this book, we will explore chakras as they make their journey across the globe, eventually making it to the west where they now stand as a key component to many spiritual world views. New Age, magical, Christianity and even some more scientific worldviews have accepted the concept of chakras into their pantheon.

The idea of chakras can work on two distinct levels according to your beliefs. Many cultures accept that these energetic centers are actual physical and subtle energetic hotspots located around our bodies. These centers act as bridges between the spiritual and physical realms. For those who do not believe in spiritual models, the chakra systems can act as a symbolic philosophy that encompasses all of our experiences as humans. Either way, these systems have to organize and enhance our day to day lives by giving us a perspective on our own existence, if not literally affecting it through spiritual or energetic work.

This book does not intend to change your religion or world view. Our intention is to explore the concepts of chakras and give you, the reader, a comprehensive guide to these ancient philosophies. As we explore these concepts, you can make your own decisions about how you use the chakra system to improve your life. It is a common misconception that chakras are specific to a certain religion, but this isn't particularly true. At this point in our world, the use of chakras is open minded enough to adhere to any worldview or religion.

Chakras are not a gift form a certain god or deity. They are naturally occurring aspects of every human's existence, simply another aspect of our bodies. It has been established that humans are electromagnetic in nature, but there is some scientific evidence that supports the idea that some parts of our bodies vibrate at different frequencies than others. This very well could be the foundational science needed to prove that chakras are literal centers of energy located throughout our bodies.

While the spiritual side of the chakra concepts goes back millennia, modern science is just now beginning to even consider the ideas as feasible. If these two worlds were to combine and support the ideas of chakras, it would validate what so many wise men and women of past centuries were teaching. Until then, we must decide for ourselves by exploring these concepts on a personal level and seeing where they lead us.

There are plenty of books on this subject on the market, thanks again for choosing this one! Every effort was made to ensure it is full of as much useful information as possible. Enjoy!

Chapter 1: Chakras and Their Origins

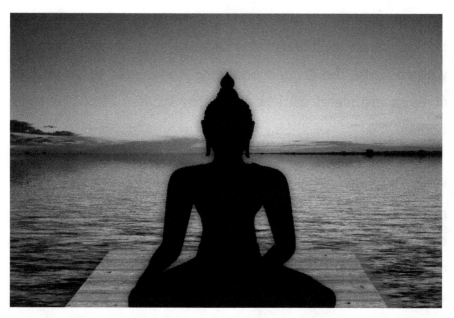

The spiritual communities in the west are greatly influenced by Catholicism and Christianity, but there are many other religious and spiritual ideas that mix and meld in the west, especially in the United States. Many of these spiritual communities accept practices like yoga and meditation but leave the philosophical topics as their own. Focusing on these powerful physical practices, these spiritual communities miss to adopt the symbolism and myth, which is left abandoned. Chakras seem to be permeating this barrier with the ideas held true by many people in Indian and the Far East.

Chakras are welcomed by many spiritual adherents who find the ideas helpful in grasping the relationship between the physical and the spiritual. We see Christianity and chakras working together most prominently in New Age communities as they mix and match practices from many cultures to create their young spiritual communities. The New Age movement may be known for an abundance of frauds and false teachers, but it has still played a great role in introducing eastern concepts with western conservative beliefs. Chakras are a great example of this.

The concept of chakras can be viewed in two ways: They can be seen as a symbolic way to organize our life experiences and examine them, or, on the other hand, they can be viewed as actual energetic centers that bridge the gap between the physical and spiritual bodies. As we explore these concepts, remember to keep an open mind. For our intents and purposes with this book, we will adhere to the idea that chakras are both of these views. They are great symbolism, but also they are actual energetic centers that can be personally worked with.

The ancient concept of chakras recognizes that chakras are energetic centers found in our subtle spiritual body. This is a further disambiguation of the concept that we all have of our physical bodies that are twinned by a subtle energetic or spiritual body. Chakras act as a means in which our physical bodies interact and influence our spiritual bodies.

Many communities in the modern age have accepted that energy is key to understanding our life experiences. Science has proven that humans are electromagnetic in nature, and this energy moves and adapts to changes in our emotional state or environment. These scientific breakthroughs are related to chakras as a means to physically feel the energy we give off or that others give off. Consider anytime you've gotten a bad vibe from someplace or someone.

The subtle energetic body needs to be cared for just as our physical body does. This is where chakra work comes into play. It is thought that chakras get blocked or closed, and we can actively work with these blockages, helping to maintain their health and consistent flow of energy between the physical and the spiritual worlds. Most traditions consider a certain chakra to be associated with a certain aspect of life, each chakra having different governance over its attributed aspects.

It is thought that there are over 80,000 different chakras throughout our bodies, claiming influence over the most subtle experiences, even experiences that we can't even feel or recognize. Most traditions do not see it worthwhile to work directly with individual chakras that are small or minuscule; so many texts are only focused on a handful of more important chakras. The main chakras are usually numbered between four and seven, respectively. With the complexity of human experience, it only makes sense that there are thousands of subtle energetic centers surrounding our bodies, not unlike the thousands of subtle autonomous occurrences that transpire in our body every moment that we physically feel.

The main chakras are much easier to notice, having a greater impact on our day-to-day lives and aspects that we constantly pay attention to. The main chakra model found in the west is the seven chakra model. These seven main chakras are recognized as the most important energetic centers in most contemporary traditions. These seven chakras are thought to encompass all aspects of our lives, from emotional experience, physical ailments, and spiritual awareness. Depending on how healthy our chakras are, these experiences can be favorable or detrimental, and in turn, affect the chakras as well, creating a cycle of energetic flow that influences our lives in incredible ways.

There may be thousands of small minuscule chakras, but these energy centers are more difficult to work with than the larger more influential chakras, that are recognized by spiritual communities and some scientific communities alike. It is worth mentioning, that it has been shown that many of the energetic pathways that our far away ancestors adhered to, actually match the nerve pathways throughout our bodies.

The ancient cultures that worked with chakras fully believed that humans lived simultaneously in the physical world and the subtle energetic world. The physical is more easy to study than the metaphysical or energetic. In fact, the physical can be observed and studied in a laboratory setting. On the other hand, the energetic world is much more abstract and unpredictable. Some people look at the physical as the only component of life. This approach is way too simplistic to encompass all of our experiences, including consciousness, perception, and other phenomena which cannot be explained or proven by science.

The main chakras will be our point of focus in this book, just as it was for our oldest ancestors. We will work to master the practices that allow us to interact directly with the chakras, thus altering our lives for the better.

We will see how these essential bridges between the physical and the spiritual world can sometimes get blocked or closed. The reasons can be different; it can be due to emotional problems, mental unbalance, and even physical ailments. Through the techniques in this book, we will learn to help our chakras stay healthy and flowing consistently.

We have now loosely defined what the chakras are, but we need to continue exploring the history and meaning of these incredible energy centers. Getting to know as much as we can about the history of chakras will help us better understand how the concepts have evolved into what they are today, how they work, and how to work with them. Simply finding the most recent source of chakras information could very well be flawed in many ways. By learning the etymology and history of these concepts, we can develop a personal practice that suits our needs, and develop our own personal views and opinions on these ancient concepts. How everyone else thinks about chakras may not fit into your perception, and of course, certain practices that work for others may not work for you. You need to develop a relationship with chakras that is personal to yourself, letting some (if not all) the practices we will discuss in this book transform your life for the better. This personalization will go a long way to further your practice and let it grow to reach your desired goals.

Etymology

Before directing towards the more practical part of the book, it is worth spending a few words on the etymology behind the concept of chakras.

The word chakra itself can be translated loosely to mean 'wheel'. This is because of the circular shape of chakras and the idea that they spin when opened or healthy. Many believe that when the chakras are closed or blocked, they do not spin at all or will spin in the opposite direction. These wheels need our attention and support to remain open and operating. This will allow the subtle energetic aspects of our lives to influence our physical ones. Such a symbiotic relationship is key in most eastern traditions and is very popular in India. These cultures heavily rely on the concept of chakras to organize and prioritize their lives, not to mention to access a world of healing outside of the modern medical sphere.

Chakras are attributed to certain physiological conditions that many humans face. Hormone production, nervous system ailments, organ health, and more generally, any other condition can be attributed to a certain chakra. Therefore, if someone is experiencing a problem in the physical world, working with the attributed chakra could help to fix the issue on a metaphysical level. Essentially, this is energy work: by healing ourselves energetically, we can heal ourselves physically.

This is not all. There are other attributes to chakras outside of the medical sphere as well. Each chakra contains many attributes associated with the physical world and our experiences as humans. Seed syllables are assigned to chakras, and these are ancient primal sounds used for mantras or meditation. Each chakra also has a color attribute, and if a chakra is blocked, the attributed color will help to open it, and keep the energy flowing. There are musical keys related to chakras, each one helping its attributed chakra by being exposed to the sound. Stones, herbs, symbols, organs, but also illnesses are all associated with a certain chakra as their energetic center. These attributes can be viewed as symbolic or actual attributes of the chakras.

On a symbolical level, we can work with the chakras through meditation to heal our minds. On a physical level, the chakras will open when aligned with the above mentioned attributes.

These interactions work on many levels and are hard to pinpoint with scientific analysis. However, either way, these practices work and can and should be utilized in our day to day lives.

It is safe to say that any interaction you have in your daily life affects your chakras in either a positive or negative way. This is where mindfulness will come into play. We need to navigate our lives in the most efficient manner to lead a fulfilling and enjoyable existence. By being aware of our surroundings and our choices, we can find our way through the world with ease. Chakras can lead us to achieve this by helping us organize our experiences and make mindful decisions each and every day. By taking the time to analyze all of our decisions through a "chakra lens", we can find paths through our chaotic world that we may not otherwise see.

Cultural Uses

Much of what we know about chakras in the west is predominantly influenced by Hinduism and Buddhist thought. These philosophies are very popular in these cultures and are used throughout the variety of religions and spiritual practices. There are also many other cultures that adhere to the idea of a spiritual body interacting simultaneously with our physical world. As an example, in Traditional Chinese Medicine, we find acupuncture and acupressure, which adhere to the concepts that there are energetic lay lines throughout the body that can be worked with.

Other cultures also adhere to the idea of an energetic presence. Almost every ancient culture owns in one form or the other the idea of the existence of a connecting energetic web. A form of energy which links all living things and beings, and which is also how we interact with the world in the nonphysical. In this book, we will center our focus on the eastern philosophies, mainly on the Indian influence and culture. As above-mentioned, the concept of chakras does not require any religion, but these concepts do stem from religious cultures. Hence, we must familiarize ourselves with their origins to be able to approach these ideas with respect and humility.

Chakra Working Basics

As we continue our exploration of the origins of chakras, we need to also touch on the very basics of how the chakra practices work. These practices vary from culture to culture. Many cultures believe that we must turn on our chakras to begin working with them. This is often symbolized as a dormant energy at the base of the spine that needs to be awakened. This dormant energy is known as Kundalini, the serpent, or snake, that guides energy up down the spine.

To awake these energies, we must be balanced both physically and energetically. The chakra energy is very concentrated and needs to be approached with patience and an open mind. Even the slightest bit of work with chakras can cause dramatic changes, this is known as a Kundalini awakening and it is not recommended that we awaken this energy in any other way except with a balanced practice and hard work.

Short cuts and use of drugs for these reasons almost always have detrimental repercussions. Opening the chakras takes dedication and determination. Depending on how blocked your chakras are, it could even take years to get the energy flowing. On the other hand, this is not a written rule, some people have documented their personal experience, with their chakras being opened in only a matter of weeks.

Despite the growing attention towards the concept of chakras and the rise in popularity, still today, the nature of chakras has yet to be fully understood, parts of it still remaining in mystery.

These energy centers truly are unique to each individual, and it is up to us to develop our own personal practice and determine what goals we are trying to reach through this practice. We have learned what chakras are and how they work, but what about their history and variety of practice from one culture to another?

The concept of chakras can be dated back to the first use of the word, but the ideas most certainly predate the written word. Even if they were yet to be called chakras, these concepts have existed in many cultures throughout history. These energetic models of reality and the true nature of the unseen forces that we interact with is at the core of every spiritual practice.

The actual use of the word chakra is first found in the Vedas, one of the most important texts in the Hindu culture. Many religions and spiritual models have sprung from these ancient texts, some using chakras some that do not. The way we define chakras today was not found in these texts. Chakras were used more like an intensive visualization tool that had a more mysterious origin than we know today.

The Vedas contained and invaluable expanse of esoteric knowledge that has now touched almost every popular religion we know. They were defined as the "king that turns the wheel of the empire", moving in every direction from a center point. We see here the related symbolism of the chakra wheels. There is also the idea of the Vedic fire altar, where there are five symbols used for visualization. These symbols were the triangle, square, circle, crescent moon, and dumpling. These shapes are also used today for chakra visualization and mandalas.

The concept of the dormant energy at the base of the spine is found in the Vedas as well, namely the Rigveda. This story tells of a yogi named Kunamnama, which is literally translated as "she who is coiled". This energy is known today as Kundalini, but the story of Kunamnama is the earliest reference to the dormant serpent energy at the base of every human's spine. This energy is known to travel the spine from its base to the base of the skull. It travels along a pathway known as Nadis.

These concepts are first found in the Upanishads form the 1st millennium BCE. Here we see the appearance of the modern chakra system, even if, for the most part we see only four main chakras with these older systems, as compared to the seven found in contemporary times. It is difficult to pin down the exact origins of the seven chakra model, but it is safe to assume that it progressively formed as the different chakra systems traveled throughout the east and made its way west, adopting new ideas and evolving into what we know it as today.

Energy models like the ones to which we adhere to today can be found since the 8th century, in Buddhist texts. These texts included chakra concepts, some earlier texts referencing vortexes that were energetic nature, although the texts do not explore them in detail. Prana and Nadi are also found during this era but lack exact origin in the texts. These words have become powerful and common in our current society with or without exact historical context, as if they have minds of their own, moving throughout the timeline right into modern times.

Buddhist texts seem to have the most influential documentation of the chakra model as we know it. Certainly, there are precursors to these texts, but the Buddhist practices concentrated heavily on these ideas, giving way to the practices we know today. The Buddhists found that there are four main chakras, these were named as Manipura, Anahata, Vishuddha and Ushnisha. These names can be loosely translated into English as Navel, heart, throat, and crown. This was often seen as spiritual counterparts to our human experiences and emotions, or the physical self twinned by the energetic or spiritual self. These ideas sparked many varying sects of Buddhist thought be split off into a variety of traditions, many that are still teaching today.

One the tradition, the Tibetan sect of Buddhism, takes the chakra models and uses the ideas of Prana and Nadis as a means to balance one's life. At the core of Tibetan Buddhism, there is the idea that learning to control the Prana through breath work, manipulating it to move through the Nadis, was the central most important practice used to reach unity with the universe. This is akin to the Kundalini energy found in Hinduism, as both models aim to reach an enlightened state through the use of energetic centers in and around our bodies.

Hindu tantric traditions are more closely related to the modern system of chakras. These traditions adhere to the Seven Chakra System, mainly inspired by hatha yoga. There are many differing views on the chakra tradition within Hinduism, but the Seven Chakra System if the most prominent and obviously the main tradition that made its way to the west.

The chakra models in Hinduism developed alongside the popular religion of Shaktism. Shakti is the premiere goddess in Hindu and other Indian traditions. The kundalini energy is even attributed to Shakti in many traditions. The chakras as energy centers are found in this system, with almost any Shakti based system adhering to the Seven Chakra System.

Death

When it comes to death within these systems, we need to consider the idea of reincarnation as the most widely practiced belief system. The idea that death is not the end of life itself, but a transgression into many other worlds. It is thought that the soul or spirit of someone may travel extensively before returning to Earth if they return at all.

In the chakra system if a person dies, their energy would leave the body behind, traveling without the body's restraints. There are a number of places this energy may travel. Many believe it returns to a source, then may leave there as well. This is similar to the idea of what this energy does when we sleep as well. Many eastern traditions believe that when we sleep, our energy is turned inward, traveling through dream-like realms. We catch glimpses of these journeys in dreams or astral projection practices.

This gives rise to questions of the physical body versus the spiritual. Many people may believe that our physical bodies are not important and that we should focus mostly on our spirit progress. In reality, while we are living with our physical bodies, we need to take great care for them as well. The physical and the energetic exist as one as far as the earthly experience is concerned. We need to care for our entire being, as we know it, to achieve our desired results.

The many chakra systems that are found throughout history are interrelated in many complex ways.

It is obvious that these concepts have borrowed from each other, melding together to form the systems we know today, including the Seven Chakra System that is so popular in the west. These systems have been at the core of many eastern traditions, and as the west accepts this ancient knowledge even more of the population begins to work with these systems, mixing them with their own practices and creating the chakra systems we know today.

Chapter 2: The Seven Chakra System

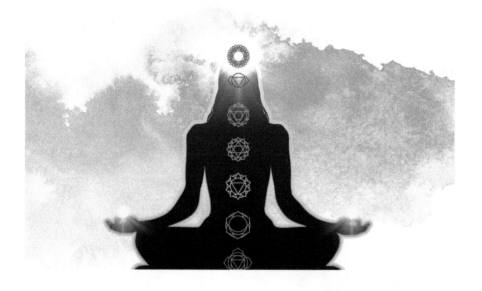

Now that we have seen the long journey that these chakra models have taken from the east into the west, evolving and influencing other cultural traditions, is the moment to focus on one of the main systems: The Seven Chakra System.

Many traditions have differing opinions about which chakras are the most important, but overall, one system has become the most widely accepted model in the west.

The Seven Chakra System finds its roots in the Vedic texts and early Buddhist texts. Evolving as it journeys westward; it has found its place as the most popular chakra system in the world. The earliest known text containing a version of a seven chakra model is dated to the 11th century. This particular model had six core chakras and a center or hub chakra at the crown, or just above the head. This system was first translated into English in the 20th century, showing how in only a short amount of time this system infiltrated the western regions.

It is most common to find the Seven Chakra System being used as symbolic meditation aids. Usually, in these circumstances, workings start at the base chakra near the bottom of the spine, working upward to the top of the head. This symbolic visualization of a spiritual evolution aims to enlighten the student, giving insight and knowledge that cannot be found elsewhere.

Kundalini

In both Buddhist and Hindu traditions, the Seven Chakra System shares the same conception, which sees the chakras pierced by the dormant energy at the base of the spine once awakened. This energy is known as Tummo in the Buddhist traditions and Kundalini in the Hindu cultures. The latter is the term which has prevailed as the preferred name in western circles. This energy is often symbolically referred to and visualized as a serpent. The serpent is thought to climb through the chakras, up the spine to the third eye.

There are many different chakra models, some of them being a reinterpretation of the Seven Chakra System.

We need to consider the influence of western culture on the seven chakra model. New Age groups and various other spiritual communities have gladly accepted these powerful practices into their circles, mixing the methods with their own views. For our purposes in this book we will stay focused on the seven chakra model that is popular in the west. We also do not affiliate with any particular religion. It is best practice to be open to everyone's ideas and world views. With that in mind, note that the seven chakra system is not biased toward any particular religion.

In the seven chakra system we have seven main chakras. This system acknowledges that there are other chakras, but they may be too subtle to work with or even feel. The seven key chakras are thought to be energy centers that pertain to all the many aspects of our lives. These energy centers are listed from the base of the spine to the crown, or area just above the head. The most accepted western system claims that we must work our way through the lowest chakra to the highest chakra, opening all of the chakras along the way. The seven main chakras are:

- Root Chakra
- Sacral Chakra
- Solar Plexus Chakra
- Heart Chakra
- Throat Chakra
- Third Eye Chakra
- Crown Chakra

Although we are engaging with these chakras naturally throughout our lives, they can become blocked or unbalanced due to general wear and tear as life progresses. If we do not tend to our chakras needs, they will become unbalanced and manifest troubles in our physical lives. No aspect of life goes untouched by our subtle energetic bodies, we must try to balance all aspects to find true healing.

Minor Chakras

It is thought that there are tens of thousands of chakras, most of them so small that we cannot even feel them. Since these chakras are so miniscule they are not actively worked with in the seven chakra system. It makes sense that there are so many minor chakras, adding complexity to the concept itself. This added complexity is similar to the complexities of life, many miniscule variables at work, but the major events are what we focus on.

The minor chakras are thought to be numbered into the tens of thousands, some traditions teaching there are up to 88,000. Some of the more prominent small chakras include the bindu, talu and manas chakras. The bindu is the most common, sometimes even being utilized in some new age circles. The bindu is often symbolically represented in some Indian cultures by wearing a jewel or crystal on their foreheads. This jewel is also known as a bindi, it is often mistaken to represent the third eye, this is a common western misconception.

The immeasurable number of minor chakras are of no concern to the beginner on the chakra path, they are reserved for more advanced study as you develop your awareness of these subtle energies. Working with minor chakras takes an even greater attention to detail, typically being focused on very specific aspects of our lives. Counting the actual number of chakras is impossible, the relationship between our subtle energetic bodies and our physical bodies is very complex, so naturally there are thousands of chakras at work.

Nadis

The concept of nadis is another concept we need to familiarize ourselves with to understand how the seven chakra system works. The energy flows through the nadis as it travels form chakra to chakra. These energetic highways are the means in which kundalini energy can find its way to the various chakras. The energy grows in intensity at certain points along the nadis, this is thought to be where the physical and subtle body meet, also known as the chakras.

Nadis are a crucial part of the energetic model that Hinduism relies upon for existential understanding. The concept of nadis is well over 3,000 years old. It is taught that there are 300,000 or more nadis that make up our energetic and physical bodies. Many believe that these nadis, channel energy to each and every cell in our body. This huge number of nadis is similar to the large number of chakras, there are thousands, but also there is a small group of prominent ones that are much more noticeable when we are working with them.

There are three main nadis that are thought to be the most important to our bodies; Ida, Pingala and Sushumna. These energetic pathways are very important in chakra work as they are the roads that our energy travels upon, building with intensity as they reach the chakra centers and moving in between the physical and energetic bodies.

The nadis are often compared to the arteries, veins and nerves that are working constantly in our bodies. The nadis are seen as the subtle energetic twin to our physical nervous system that carries physical nutrients and oxygen throughout our bodies. These comparisons are becoming more popular as science reveals the mysterious nature of the human body and its energetic capabilities. It is safe to say that all physical aspect of our lives has a counterpart in the energetic body.

When we are working with our chakras we must take into consideration the nadis and how the energy is able to move. Working with the nadis allows us to easily move blockages, if we only focus on the chakras we have no means of moving the blockages, without these energetic channels our energy cannot flow consistently. This is similar to Chinese models that adhere to the idea of meridian lines throughout the body. It is believed that these meridian lines can become blocked if not properly cared for, we can safely assume that the meridian lines and nadis are identical concepts. Let's explore the *Ida*, *Pingala* and *Sushumna* nadis in more details.

Ida

The energetic channel called *Ida* is associated with lunar energy and feminine energy. It has a cooling effect and is the channel for creative energy. This energy is nurturing and fluid, often changing erratically if left to its own devices. This channel is also known as an introverted energy, stimulating deep thought and self-analysis.

Pingala

The energetic channel called *Pingala* is associated with solar energy and masculine energy. It has a warming effect and is the channel for reasoning and logic. This energy promotes survival tactics and offers a fiery motivation that can often get out of control if left unchecked. Extroverted energy is associated with this channel, stimulating social interaction and the drive to accomplish our goals.

Ida and Pingala Relationship

The *Ida* and *Pingala* are thought to be two parts of a whole. These energetic channels are the two main channels in the seven chakra system, making up the main channels that the chakra energy travels through. Some traditions teach that *Ida* and *Pingala* crisscross each other at the chakras, switching places on either side of the middle channel, *Sushumna*. Other traditions teach that *Ida* and *Pingala* always run along their respected side of the body, the *Ida* on the left and the *Pingala* on the right. These channels run from the lower body near the genitalia, up to the third eye chakra where they do cross *Sushumna* then exit through the nostrils. It is thought that our breath helps to carry this energy along the nadis, then out of our bodies on the breath.

Being able to control our breathing is crucial for our purposes in this book. The power of breathing is thought to be a life force that helps to move energy and heal our bodies. If our breath is inconsistent or too short, we can cause blockages in our chakras. By taking control of our breathing we can balance our energetic body and calm our physical selves as well. Consider anytime you've been nervous or afraid, your breath becomes shorter and inconsistent, as if you are gasping for air. This is the natural way our breathing changes when we are in danger or upset, but if we breathe through it, we find that deep slow breaths actually calm our minds and our physical nerves.

Ida and *Pingala* are often symbolized as the two hemispheres of the brain. The popular concept that the right and left sides of our brain govern different human experiences is common in the western society. Many claim that the right brain is the dictator of creativity and spontaneity, while the left side is the governor of reason and problem solving. It needs to be noted that many ancient cultures have similar concepts.

Sushumna

The energetic channel called *Sushumna* runs directly through the middle of the spine. It's generally viewed as starting at the root chakra then running up to the crown chakra, culminating at the other chakras along the way. This is the main channel that *Ida* and *Pingala* are guided by. *Suchumna* is the middle path, it is unchanging and less fluid than *Ida* and *Pingala*. All nadis are said to connect to *Sushumna* in some way, it is the main channel of travel for our body's energy. The main highway. This channel acts as a hub for all other nadis. During a kundalini awakening many people express that they can feel the power of *Sushumna* more so than any other nadi.

Similar concepts of nadis and the philosophy attributed to them are found throughout many cultures; the balance of female and male energies, lunar and solar energies, or watery and fiery energies. These concepts are popular as yin and yang in eastern philosophies, and it seems the west has adopted this concept as well. It is thought that the feminine and masculine energies are the main energetic properties that make up all the other subtle energies.

Balancing the masculine and feminine energies requires an overall balanced lifestyle. Physically and energetically we must remain balanced to get the most out of our energetic work. This means intentionally engaging the logical masculine energy and the creative feminine energy. With overstimulation of one or the other, we find that we cannot lead fulfilling lives. Keep this in mind when approaching your chakra practices.

Now we can see the seven chakra system taking form, with energetic channels crisscrossing all throughout our being, forming potent energetic centers we now know as chakras. This complex system may seem overwhelming at first, but with just a little work and dedication, we can familiarize ourselves with the system and work with it to improve our lives.

With the added nadis, or pathways, of *Ida*, *Pingala* and *Sushumna* we learn how each chakra can interact with each other, and further move throughout our bodies. It is easy to now visualize how these paths can become blocked, not unlike a busy highway. To maintain these paths we must act as creator and repair our energetic roads, making sure to maintain them throughout our lives, or face the illness and troubles that accompany blockages.

As we continue, take time to learn these attributes and how they may interact with your life. Memorize the attributes, the colors, sounds and concepts, fully to help you properly engage with the chakras as we move on to the practice section of the book.

Chapter 3: Chakra Unbalance

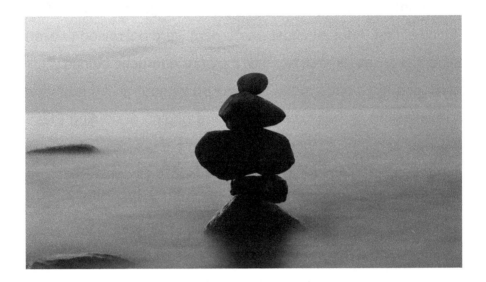

We have seen that our chakras can become unbalanced or blocked, but what does this feel like? Is it something we can readily feel on a day to day basis? These energetic centers are very subtle, and any unbalance or blockage can be hard to notice at first. After all, most westerners were not raised to even accept chakras as real, nor that they are energetic beings. This misconception leads many to grow up without giving attention to the feeling of their own energy and ending attributing these feelings to other sources. There is no shame in not being mindful of chakras as a beginner. Some people are more perceptive and naturally inclined to recognize and work on and with their energy. Differently, others need to work a bit harder to achieve the necessary skills to feel and work with their energy. Whichever your case is, please keep in mind that anyone can learn to work with and feel their chakras.

Some traditions believe that everything in your life is related to chakras and their balance. This may be true in some sense, but we also need to consider the existence of other variables which are at work as well. The first logical step is to focus on the signs which tell us that our chakras are unhealthy. These signs can manifest in our personal lives and physical bodies. Lack of energy, trouble sleeping, unbalanced appetite, depression, and many other common symptoms can arise from unbalanced and blocked chakras. Let's explore these ailments in detail and learn how to tell if our chakras are unbalanced.

Subtle Energy

If you were raised in the west, chances are, you have not worked with your chakras at all your entire life. This more than likely means your chakras could use a little love. Since the energy flowing through any human being is so subtle, it can be difficult, especially at the beginning to pinpoint its effects. Consider any time you had strange feelings for no reason or woke up feeling bad. These feelings that seem to have no source usually can be related to energetic blockages or uncomfortable energy around you. Learning to recognize and work with these subtle energies is key to developing a fruitful chakra practice.

When trying to learn whether or not your chakras are unbalanced, it is good to start with noticeable aspects of your life that are causing trouble. If you have some specific ailments that are debilitating, consider which chakra may be related to that ailment and work on that chakra to see if you experience any relief. Keep in mind that ailments do not necessarily have to be physical problems; they can very much be emotional troubles or personal things that you wish to improve.

When analyzing your life to see what aspects need the most attention, it can be helpful to start a journal to keep track of your progress. Begin by taking the time to list the aspects of your life you wish to improve. These can be physical aspects or emotional aspects. You may even want to list aspects of your life that you wish to improve which aren't related to your body or emotions. You may want to list things such as your financial status or environment. Make a comprehensive list and be truthful to yourself.

Once you have your list of ailments ready, you can go through it and prioritize its content. You have to organize it by which aspects need to be improved immediately and which ones can be focused on in the future. This list is the starting point to create a structure for our chakra practice, focusing on the parts of our life that need attention the most.

Eventually, we will associate each of these problems to the specific chakra they pertain to. Take time to see if you can write this list and organize it into seven categories one for each chakra we learned about in the previous chapter. Some aspects will be easy to categorize according to chakra, while others may be difficult to assign a chakra to. Some issues may need to be assigned to two or three different chakras.

Do your best to organize your list by chakra. You may even wish to use the attributed colors to make sure your list is clear. It is ok if you cannot categorize them yet, as we will be looking at each chakra in detail in due course.

If you have been truthful to yourself, going through the list, you will notice that there is much work to do to achieve your desired goals. It is important that you do not feel overwhelmed by the size of this list. In fact, you will soon realize that once you start solving certain problems other issues will begin to balance out as well. Since all aspects of life are interlinked your progress in one aspect of life will most certainly affect the different areas of your existence.

Unbalanced Chakra Exercise

We have learned about the Seven Chakra System and which chakras may relate to certain aspects of our lives. As we begin to see our practice forming, we also need to start to learn how to feel our chakras. The following exercise is a simple beginner's exercise to help develop your sensitivity to chakra energy.

Don't worry if you struggle visualizing the chakras at this stage. The following chapters will cover each individual chakra in detail. While you proceed with your reading remember to come back to this exercise to continue your practice.

Exercise:

To begin this exercise, you need to find a quiet place where you can sit down and not be distracted. You will need at least thirty uninterrupted minutes to spend alone to complete this exercise.

Once you have found a comfortable seated position, take the time to focus on your breathing and relax. Clear your mind, let your thoughts roll by, make sure not to get caught up on any of them.

Once you have found a reasonably peaceful state, it is time to start visualizing your chakras. Begin with the root chakra and move up all the way up to the crown chakra before moving back down to the root.

Don't rush, take the time to stop at each chakra. Visualize its color, and try to feel its position in relation to your spine and body.

As you continue to visualize the chakras, take a mental note of any particular chakra which stands out to you. If you feel any blockages or uncomfortable feelings when focusing on a specific chakra, you will know that one may need your attention to unblock and clear it.

Focus on raising your awareness in regards to any anomalies you experience while visualizing the chakras. Attempt to breathe through them as you focus on your chakras. Take deep breaths as you move from chakra to chakra. You may even want to use your hands to try and feel the energy flowing through the chakra as well.

Understandably, many beginners find it difficult to feel the chakras. Do not get discouraged if the first few times you do not perceive much. As you practice the techniques explained in this book, you will gradually improve, and finally, you will obtain the results you are aiming for.

Practice is the key which will lead you to learn how to pinpoint the energy and to know how to work with it. With a little practice, you will earn how to know which of your chakras need attention, even before the energy blockages manifest in your day to day life as disruptive events.

Use this exercise as much as possible. As simple as it is, it can easily become a part of a healthy routine. Try to practice this exercise once a day for five to seven days a week. This exercise is a great way to start your day in the morning or to wind down just before bed.

As we learn to recognize our unbalanced chakras, we can begin to improve our life through a working practice with them. Having this skill is crucial to working with your chakras. Soon, you will start to notice the slightest change in the chakras' energy. During your day to day tasks, you will notice how your surroundings can affect your chakras. In fact, it is not rare for people to realize how their jobs have a detrimental effect on their chakras.

Practicing the above exercise is not only great for learning how your chakras move, but can also act a healing method for day to day wear and tear. To evolve this exercise and practice clearing your chakras, visualize white light from the heavens slowly coming down and flowing through your chakras. This is a very basic practice that can help maintain healthy chakras and clear away any recent blockages you may have accumulated that day.

Blockage Manifestation

Learning to feel the blockages in your chakras is not the only way to keep track of your chakra health. It is common for energetic blockages to cause issues throughout your surroundings, not just in your physical body. For example, if you find that you are not heard by others, or that people tend to misunderstand what you are saying, you could have a blockage in the throat chakra interfering with your communication. Alternatively, if you have problems maintaining a steady home or providing for your loved ones, a possibility is that you may have blockages in your root chakra. It is fundamental to dedicate time to recognize the role the different chakras can play in every aspect of our lives, not just our personal health.

When these energetic blockages manifest in these intensive ways, it is usually a sign that your chakras are in need of some serious help. Bear in mind that this is not uncommon in a society where the concept of natural energy is rarely accepted, and its role in our lives is not recognized. As we learn to take care of our chakras, we can better understand the true nature of our subtle energetic bodies and work with them to improve our lives.

Blockages or unbalances in your chakras can manifest in many ways. Some traditions teach that all aspects of life are a result of energetic influence. This can be helpful when trying to overcome adversity during our day to day living. If we can view our world through a chakra lens, we can see that interconnectedness of all things. This interconnectedness is key to rebuilding our relationship with our chakras. We may not be able to control all aspects of our environment, but we can control the energy we let in and put out into the world.

Chapter 4: Healing and Balancing Chakras

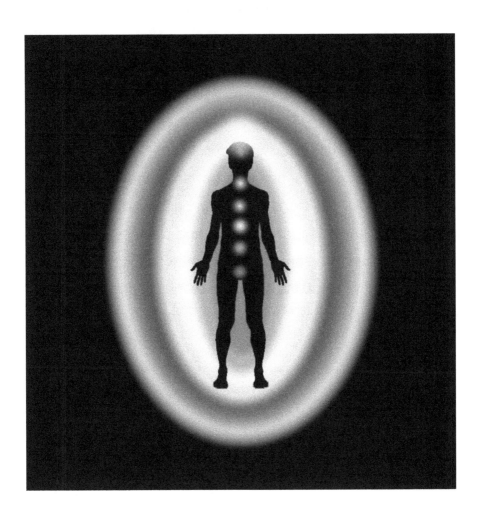

The first step on the path to a new relationship with our chakras is clearing away any blockages that have formed over the course of our lives. Since many westerners have never taken any time to think about their energetic centers, nor to take care of them, they often find that their chakras need some serious attention. Imagine a lifetime's worth of energetic blockages and unbalance accumulating in your chakras, this can cause serious issues if not taken care of.

To clear away blockages and balance the chakras is very similar to caring for any other part of your body, only it's not physical. Just like you clean your body, our chakras need a little help to clear away energetic gunk and balance the flow of energy to and from the physical and energetic worlds. Since we cannot physically scrub our chakras, we must learn some useful energy work techniques to help our chakras.

The idea that we can manipulate energy for our personal gain is an ancient one. There is no doubt that everything is energetic, science has proved this. But being able to intentionally move the energy is a skill that takes time and dedication. Imagine anytime you've walked into a room and the energy there has been uncomfortable. Maybe someone received some bad news, or the room is just energetically dense. Either way, you naturally notice this energy, you are aware of the negative situation because you can feel it. Essentially, this is what we are looking for when we look for blockages in our chakras. You may feel a similar feeling inside you during certain situations or on a regular basis throughout your day. This is an energetic blockage. Feeling it is a good thing. If you feel it, then you can target it and work with it to balance the chakra.

We have the ability to literally move the energy using our hands, but we can also visualize and move the energy using our minds. This is described as using your energy to move the blockages, like water moving a log or dam. Most of us have experienced a time when we could easily move our energy. Usually, this happens during times of emotional distress or anger. You can feel the energy seeping through your pores, and you can even extend the discomfort to others. Many call this 'bad vibes' or similar slang terms, but it is definitely authentic and very powerful.

Some people use their energetic skills to drain others, abusing their inherent powers. This can be seen as a form of vampirism or energetic attack. For our intents and purposes in this book, we are not using our energetic skills for evil. Three can be very detrimental reactions if you intentionally use your power for negative reasons. It is counterproductive to want to lead a balanced and happy life and also tear others down. These attacks are not recommended and we do not condone them .

Using your energetic skills for the greater good is the ultimate path for students who wish to work with chakra energy. As you develop your skills, you will be able to not only work on yourself, but you may even be skilled enough to work on other people. We see this energy healing in many new age communities. The practice of Reiki or energetic massage is very similar to this healing practice. The role of the healer is key to many cultures throughout history. Consider the shaman who travels to various worlds to heal the community and protect his people. Or the many people who dedicate their lives to exploring alternative healing methods when synthetic ones fail. These roles are essential to the survival of any society, but these roles have also gone lost in western culture. They have, in fact, been replaced by synthetic medicines or surgeries.

As they begin their journey working with chakras, many people are surprised to discover that they are very skilled with the practices. Those of us who are naturally skilled in these processes are the ones who will be the most successful when working to heal people and environments. There is a saying that some people are doors, and some are windows, meaning, some people are just more naturally inclined to energy work, but it is an attainable skill for everyone.

Please, always remember the importance of an open-minded approach and the essential role a positive mindset plays for you to successfully reach your goals.

When it comes to developing your skills to clear and balance chakras, there are many simple exercises that you need to practice a lot. The concept of energetic work is quite simple, but breaking our preconceived notions of reality can be difficult.

In modern society, we are raised to believe that a pill is the answer to any sort of illness. While there are circumstances where we must follow this advice, in other cases we should leave this idea behind in exchange for a more energetic and natural view of the world.

Clearing Exercise

For a simple chakra clearing exercise, we can start from the exercise explained in the previous chapter and extend it.

Once again, you need to find a quiet place where you can sit in silence and undisturbed, someplace where you will not be disrupted. You will need to sit for at least thirty minutes in peace.

Once you have our mind clear and you are not distracted by mundane thoughts, you can visualize our chakras. Then you will imagine the cleansing white light coming from the heavens. This pure light will act as clean energy to clear your chakras. Let the light pierce them one by one and then flow through them, imagine the light connecting all seven chakras.

As you breathe, imagine your exhales are carrying unwanted energy and blockages out of your body. When you inhale be sure not to bring them back in. Do this for as long as you see fit, letting the light cleanse your entire energetic being. It is important that you stay focused during this practice, do not let your thoughts interfere with your cleansing practice.

This is a relatively simple practice to get you started. We will cover more in depth practices to heal the chakras as well. There are many ways to help balance your chakras, including using sound, color, yoga, meditation, foods, and an abundant array of other practices.

Chakra Movement

When clearing and balancing chakras, we need to take into consideration the way that they move. We have learned that chakras are circular or disc-shaped, it is now time to focus on the fact that this is not only the chakras' shape, it is also the way these energy centers move, like discs.

Most traditions teach that the chakras are spinning, almost like a vortex or whirlpool. When chakras are blocked, they will not be able to spin at all. In fact, if they become completely closed, they will not move at all. If you do not feel a certain chakra moving, then it may very well be closed or blocked.

Some traditions claim that a chakra will move clockwise or counter clockwise depending on the health of the chakra. This motion is very difficult to feel. So, for the intent of this book, as a general rule, if your chakras are moving, it's a good sign.

When we visualize our chakras, we can visualize the circular motion they make, this will help us know how to work with any given chakra depending on how it moves. If you feel intense movement near a certain chakra, then it is more than likely healthy. We are seeking balance here, so we do not want to overstimulate a chakra either. If it's moving, then it's best to focus on other chakras that may be blocked.

As we further our practice, we need to take an in depth look at each chakra and at its attributes. It is recommended that you build a relationship with each individual chakra, learning its behavior and attributes. This will help you recognize which chakra needs your attention. Eventually, you will reach a stage where you are able to feel which ones of your chakras need balancing.

Practice the beginner's techniques you have learned so far to help you build relationships with each chakra. As we begin to learn about each chakra individually, use these exercises to explore each individual chakra.

This is an ongoing process, so you need to spend as much time as possible practicing these exercises. This is the only way you will familiarize with your chakras and become aware of what their needs are.

Chapter 5: The Root Chakra

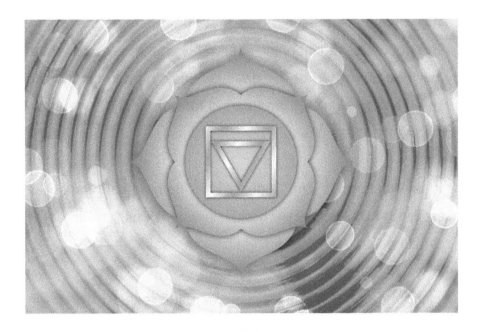

The root chakra is the chakra located at the base of the spine. This is often referred to as the first chakra. It is the most primal chakra and typically is attributed to primordial behavior or animal-like characteristics. The official name of this chakra, *Muladhara*, which comes from the words *"Mula"*, which means root and *"Dhara"*, which means support.

Muladhara

The root chakra pertains to primal needs of humans and the basics of survival. It is located at the base of the spine, governing the essential of life itself. This chakra is represented by our needs instead of our desires. Basic human functioning such as eating, drinking, and caring for our family are the key components of this chakra.

If it is blocked, it can manifest in detrimental ways like overeating, homelessness, broken relationships, and in some circumstances, even through violent outbreaks.

Working through this chakra requires us to take control of our essential needs and engage with them in healthy ways. Healthy eating, caring for family or ancestors, and taking care of our earthly problems are all great ways to open this chakra.

This area is also where the Kundalini serpent energy sleeps, coiled dormant until it is awakened through chakra exercises and practices. It is important to address here that a Kundalini awakening is an intensive experience, and if not handled with the utmost can cause detrimental effects. Approaching complex breathwork or other exercises without the required experience can lead to a premature release of this energy, causing trauma or even mental issues. It is recommended that you approach these practices patiently, forming a balanced practice, and putting in the hard work needed to reach these goals in a healthy way.

The root chakra is symbolized by a four-petaled lotus flower with a triangle pointed downward within a square at its center. Breaking away from our primal nature and working toward a more loving and compassionate nature is key to opening this chakra. Instead of selfish or individualist behavior, we can practice unconditional love. We need to utilize our primal instincts as well, ensuring to give importance to our survival. This is a delicate balance that is very important to working with the chakras. We must utilize all the chakras to achieve our desired goals. They work together to create what we know as the self, maintaining the balance of these aspects is our primary goal in this book.

The root chakra governs our most animalistic behaviors. Fear, survival, but also procreation are all greatly influenced by this chakra. The health of this chakra heavily influences our ability to maintain shelter and provide for ourselves and our families. If our root chakra is unbalanced or blocked, we may find ourselves without shelter or a healthy home life. We may not be in control of our animal instincts with an unbalanced root chakra as well. This may manifest in a variety of ways including unhealthy sex life, bad diet, bad personal hygiene, and the externalization of childish or immature behavior.

The root chakra is the foundation of the chakra system. If we cannot balance our most basic and primal instincts, then we are not going to be able to efficiently work with the higher chakras. Without shelter, food, and family, we cannot truly begin to get a grip on a balanced lifestyle. These are the building blocks of a fulfilling life, and they are the foundation of our existence and should be taken very seriously.

The root chakra is often overlooked by those who seek only spiritual revelation when working with the seven chakras system. It is a common mistake to undermine the root chakra as being primal, or not important to spiritual development. This is a terrible mistake. We must balance our most crucial aspects of life to even begin working with spiritual ideas. We require a strong base to build upon if we wish to gain access to higher knowledge. This is where the root chakra comes into play.

The root chakra is relatively easy to recognize when it is unbalanced. It manifests in ways that are very obvious, like family arguments or the desire to procreate and start a family. These are the very basic instincts for any human being, and they must not be ignored.

Root Chakra Blockages

There are many signs that can manifest when your root chakra is not balanced. Often these problems will manifest in the area that the chakra is located, so you may have problems with body parts below the spine. Restless legs, aching feet, and stiffness are common with this chakra's unbalance.

You may physically feel off balance if your root chakra is blocked. This can result in dizziness or tripping over your own feet often. You will have low energy and feel slowed down in your day to day actions, you may feel generally unmotivated, and you will not want to exercise.

When experiencing problems related to the root chakra, you may also feel insecure. Finances, home life, and the future may be overwhelming or causing stress in unexpected ways. These are your survival instincts telling you that your chakras are unbalanced. More often than not, your fears and perceptions related to your stability will be exaggerated when the root chakra is blocked.

Root Chakra Balancing

To balance the root the chakra you need to ground yourself, connecting to the earth for support. Eating root vegetables will help you in doing this, as well as going outside with bare feet and feeling the earth below you. Stretch outdoors with no shoes or socks on, or simply sit on the bare earth and breathe.

Have you ever walk barefoot on the beach? Have you ever felt the water around your feet? Have you ever experienced the sensation of the grass on your bare skin?

If you do, you are likely to remember the feeling of relief you have experienced. Being in contact with the ground allows us to free our energy, let go of the electromagnetic energy each human being carries. Grounding ourselves enables us to free our minds from our worries.

The color red is associated with the root chakra, so wearing red will help to stimulate and clear the chakra. You may also wish to visualize red mandalas and meditate on the images to help clear your root chakra.

Attributes

The color of the root chakra is red, we can wear red or decorate our home to stimulate the chakra.

The stone associated with this chakra is onyx. We can carry this stone in our pocket or wear it in jewelry to balance the root chakra.

The metal associated with the root chakra is lead. Lead is toxic, so it is not recommended to be used by beginners or without precautions.

The mineral associated with this chakra is calcium. We can balance out the root chakra by including more or less calcium rich foods in our diet.

The musical key for the root chakra is C. Listening to songs in this key or mediating on the C note will help to balance this chakra.

The seed sound for the root chakra is LAM. Chanting or listening to recordings of this sound can balance this chakra.

The glands associated with this chakra are the gonads.

The flavor attributed to this chakra is bitterness. Balance your diet with not too much or too little of its flavor to balance the root chakra.

Chapter 6: The Sacral Chakra

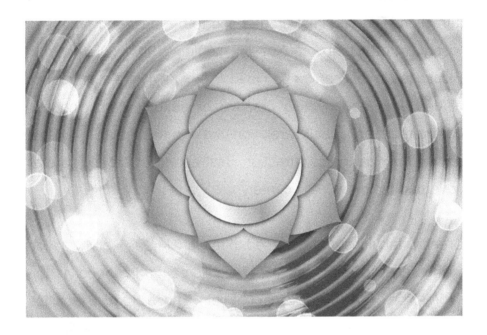

The second chakra up from the base of the spine is the sacral chakra. Known as Svadhishthana, which translated to "where the self is established" and connects us to our emotions and desires. Svadhisthana is located in the abdomen, about 2 inches below the navel. This chakra is known for the primal creative faculties of the human experience. It is associated with healthy sexual energy and the need to express your emotions in healthy ways.

Svadhishthana

This chakra is associated with sexual encounters and attraction. These primal urges need to be mastered and used wisely rather than carelessly indulging in your desires. Blockages in this chakra can lead to sexual dysfunction or lack of desire to do anything creative or sexual. Balancing this chakra requires a healthy relationship with sex, as an individual and with our partners. Attraction, desire, and procreation are all governed by this energy center.

Creative faculties are attributed to this chakra as well. Creation in the sense of procreation but also creation intended as the expression of artistic tasks or concepts. These creative faculties are attuned to the primal energy of the sacral chakra, while also being closely related with intuitive abilities of the third eye chakra. The creative process itself can be viewed as a symbolic journey through the chakras, starting at the creative source in the sacral chakra, then making its way upward as the creative processes become intuitive instead of mechanical.

The sacral chakra's image is a six-petaled lotus flower with a crescent moon at its center. The moon relates to the water element and also fertility. This chakra is fluid and ever-changing, much like expression, which can make it tough for many to balance and open. Through a balanced sex life, control of desire, and creative endeavors, this chakra can be easily managed.

While associated with primal energies similar to the root chakra, the sacral chakra's primal current is less about survival and more related to creativity and expression. There is a sense of individualism we see developing with this chakra. Our personal preferences come into play as we express ourselves through attraction, whether it is sexual attraction or simply the things we enjoy. Creativity is key to this chakra. Many may feel that they are not creative when it comes to the arts, but we must consider all types of creative endeavor. How we dress is creative, how we love is creative, how we speak is creative, and of course, through sex we create. This rhythm of life pulses through every one of us, and is the essence of the creative spirit.

If the root chakra is the foundation of the seven chakra system, then the sacral chakra is the inspiration. This inspiration motivates us and gives us reason to thrive. Indulgence and passion thrive in the sacral chakra. This chakra is often over stimulated for many who indulge in drugs, alcohol or promiscuous sex. Balancing your enjoyment of intoxicating things is key to a healthy sacral chakra.

Creating is crucial for this chakra as well. Although not all of us are painters, writers and in general artists, each person can find ways to use their creative faculties in their day to day life. Gardening, exercise, organization, self-love, companionship, and many other aspects of life can be viewed as creative in nature. Essentially, any hobby or emotional expression can be creative, so treat it as such.

Art, music, dancing, and overall anything enjoyable to the senses is heavily influenced by the sacral chakra. The arts are important aspects of all of humanity, inspiring generations to enjoy life and seek its mysteries openly. The enjoyment of the arts is one of the most unique things about humans, often the linchpin that sets us apart from other inhabitants of Earth. To find inspiration in these arts to stimulate and balance the sacral chakra.

Blockages

When your sacral chakra is blocked or unbalanced, you may feel pain or stiffness in areas on your body related to the chakra. This could manifest as pain in your lower back and hips. You may lack sexual drive or feel emotionally uninspired by things that usually excite you.

Lack of sex drive is a very common problem with sacral chakra problems. This can manifest in physically not being able to perform, or mentally being unattracted to your partner, or feeling that you are unattractive. The lack of interest in sex is very common for many middle-aged people, and simple sacral chakra exercises can help immensely with these issues.

Sacral blockages may cause you to feel a lack of creative inspiration or a sense that you are not contributing to society in a creative or important way. This loss of imagination is obvious, as your thoughts became less fantastical and more mundane. Even your dreams may be boring, consisting of only common day to day tasks.

You may also feel emotionless when your sacral chakra is unbalanced. This is very dangerous, often leading to depression or the inability to care. This numb feeling can lead to many other issues as well, often affecting other chakras in similar ways.

Balancing

To balance the sacral chakra, it is recommended to get in touch with water. Baths, swimming or a short dip in a natural body of water will help your sacral chakra to become unblocked. Dancing and other exercises that imply moving the hips do wonders for the sacral chakra as well.

The emotional problems that accompany sacral chakra blockages are a bit more complicated to work with. You may need to seek professional help from a therapist to get to the core of your emotional issues. Starting a journal will also help to analyze your emotions from an outsider's perspective.

Wearing the color orange will help balance the sacral chakra. Visualize orange mandalas, or simply immerse yourself in orange to help get the energy flowing smoothly through the sacral chakra.

Attributes

The color attributed to the sacral chakra is orange, you can wear orange or even decorate your room in orange to help balance this chakra.

The stone attributed to this chakra is beryl. You can carry this stone in your pocket or have jewelry made using this stone.

The metal of the sacral chakra is tin. You can use this metal to make jewelry or carry it with you to help balance the chakra.

The mineral of the sacral chakra is sodium. If your sacral chakra is unbalanced, you may be ingesting too much or too little of this mineral.

The musical key of the sacral chakra is D. Listening to songs in this key or meditating on the note D will help balance this chakra.

The seed sound of the sacral chakra is Vam. Chanting or meditating on recordings of this sound will help to balance the chakra.

The sexual organs are associated with this chakra. If your chakra is blocked, you may experience a lack of sexual drive or inefficient organ function.

In term of food, salty flavors are the ones attributed to the sacral chakra. If you consume too much salty food, or too little, your sacral chakra could become unbalanced.

Chapter 7: The Solar Plexus Chakra

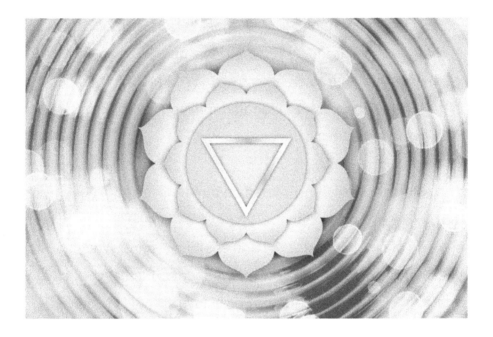

The solar plexus chakra is the third chakra up from the base of the spine and it's located above the navel or slightly below the solar plexus. It is called *Manipura*, which translates to "lustrous gem" and relates to your ability to be confident and control your life. It is the battery of our energetic body, offering the physical energy to accomplish what needs to be done. This chakra is often linked to the sun, powering all of life on earth.

Manipura

The navel chakra is known commonly as the solar plexus for its relation to the sun. This chakra is thought of as a source of energy, governing energy levels, and the ability to put in the work needed to achieve your goals. Some traditions also consider this chakra to be related to the beginning of a person's journey on the path to self-discovery. Working with this chakra is key to develop the intention and motivation to continue your path to expanded consciousness.

The solar plexus is often seen as a threshold as you move from the primal chakras near the base of the spine to the higher chakras of emotional stability and spiritual insight. Working with this chakra is crucial to find the energy and mental capacity to deal with emotions and the power of love.

The solar plexus is symbolized by a ten-petaled lotus flower, with a downward-pointing triangle at its center. The downward-pointing triangle is symbolic of fire in many elemental concepts found in many traditions. This fire is the source of energy which we all need to continue with our journey, burning out primal fears and troubles to make room for purer emotions like love and compassion.

The solar plexus chakra shines brightly, powering our bodies so that we may have the stamina and energy to navigate our lives. To seek survival and creativity found in the lower chakras, we need our battery to power our endeavors. Working for food and shelter or listening to or creating music, these tasks need power behind them to keep the gears working. The solar plexus is where we find the desire and motivation to move on throughout our days.

Just as the earth could not exist without its sun, our six other chakras cannot be stimulated and worked with without the power supplied by the solar plexus chakra. This chakra governs our energetic distribution, giving agency to the energy so it may move freely through our chakras. At the core of our being we may have primal instincts and inspirations, but moving up past our necessary survival tactics we have the energy that promotes free will and pursuit of the greater powers of the universe. The solar plexus chakra connects our primal roots to the greater pursuit.

Through the solar plexus chakra, we find a bridge from animal instinct to human compassion and love. Along with this incredible love comes free will and self-love. We take control of our emotions and move them intentionally, finding what love truly means to us and sharing it with our family, friends, and community. This is the core of human evolution and growth.

Blockages

The blockages in your solar plexus chakra can manifest in a variety of ways, including physical pain in the area where the chakra is located. Digestive issues and problems in and around the abdomen are common with the lack of balance in the solar plexus chakra.

Since this chakra is our battery, we may feel a lack of energy and motivation when it is unbalanced. This lethargic state is often attributed to laziness or lack of exercise, but the solar plexus plays a huge role as well. If this chakra is blocked, you will notice that you are not functioning efficiently in many aspects of life, lacking dedication and self-esteem.

This chakra can also be overstimulated, leading to egoism and selfish behaviors. This is not an uncommon situation. Many people who started working with the solar plexus, experienced an increase in their self-esteem. Consequently, they became more and more proud of their accomplishments to the point their ego ended up distracting them from their real intentions and goals.

Often, this selfish behavior is the cause which prevents people from continuing their path through the different chakras to arrive to the heart chakra. Selfishness can, in fact lead to a lack of commitment, loneliness and even rude behavior, such as abusing power roles at work.

Balancing

To balance the solar plexus chakra we need to connect with the fiery nature of motivation and determination. Meditating on a flame such as a candle can benefit, as well as spending time in the sunlight. Camping and other outdoor activities are perfect for the solar plexus.

Fasting and general detox is suitable for this chakra as well. Change your diet to include easily digested foods and brightly colored foods like fruits and vegetables. Yellow is associated with this chakra, so wearing yellow may help as well.

Attributes

The color of the solar plexus chakra is yellow. You can wear yellow clothing or decorate your room with yellow to help balance this chakra.

The stone of the solar plexus chakra is ruby. This stone can be carried in your pocket or worn in jewelry.

The metal of this chakra is iron. This metal can be worn as jewelry or carried with you in a pocket.

The mineral of the solar plexus chakra is sulfur. If your solar plexus chakra is unbalanced, you may be ingesting too much or too little of this mineral. Alter your diet accordingly.

The musical key of the solar plexus chakra is E. If your chakra is unbalanced, you can listen to songs in this key or meditate on the E note to balance it.

The seed sound of this chakra is Ram. Chant this sound or listen to recordings of it to balance your solar plexus chakra.

The pancreas is associated with the solar plexus chakra. If your pancreas is not functioning properly, you may have blockages in this chakra.

Pungent flavors are the ones associated with this chakra. Balance the amount of pungent flavors you include in your diet to make sure your solar plexus chakra remains healthy and balanced.

Chapter 8: The Heart Chakra

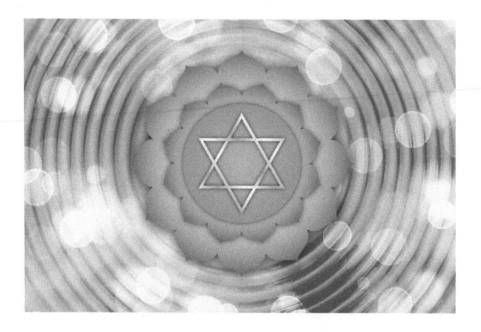

The fourth primary chakra is the Heart or *Anahata* chakra, which translates to "unhurt, unstruck, and unbeaten". The heart chakra is the chakra that governs our ability to show love and compassion toward others. This ability to love is key to human evolution and growth. Unconditional love and self-love are key components to this chakra, and knowing this great love is what truly makes the human experience unique. The heart chakra is located in the central channel of the spine near the heart.

Anahata

This chakra is key to experiencing self-love, love for others, and compassion. In traditional Buddhist models, empathy and compassion are key to spiritual growth and mindfulness. Here we see that working your way through the chakras requires great attention to these basic human emotions that are often taken for granted.

The power of love is important to connect the gap between the spiritual and the physical bodies. The role of the heart chakra is to keep these energies balanced. If we are not able to accept love or compassion, then we may have blockages in the heart chakra, or even the lower chakras, not allowing us to access the heart chakra whatsoever. It is no secret that love is the most important experience as we live our lives, many people find love or learn love, then continue their lives happily, not trying to access the higher chakras or states of being. This is perfectly fine and makes for a balanced and beautiful existence. For seekers of deeper knowledge, they take the love they know and use it to reach higher plains of thinking.

The heart chakra is symbolized by a twelve-petaled lotus with two intertwined triangles at its center. The interlocking triangles are a symbol found in many religions and spiritual concepts. Consider the Star of David or the key of Solomon in occult teachings. This symbol represents the unification of male and female, fire and water, and many times is used for protection against evil energy.

Survival, expression, and our energetic battery form a foundation for our love to grow. Being able to accept and give love is the most rewarding experience for humans. We may be able to provide for our families, but doing it with love takes honor and humility. Giving love in a selfless way is the ultimate sacrifice as you give a literal piece of yourself to others in exchange for nothing. Practicing this unconditional love is one of the most important tasks for our society to adopt. This unconditional love is what truly makes our living experience incredible. It is the most intimate way to express your affection for someone.

Living your life, sharing love in an unconditional manner is much more difficult than it may seem. Our society is based on capitalist and individualist behavior. Often our survival is based on whether or not we can outwit others. This leads to selfish behavior that leads to selfish lifestyles. Without love, these endeavors are worthless, we can gain all the material wealth we want, but nothing compares to the love that is shared unconditionally.

As we navigate our day to day lives, we are motivated by survival, inspiration, and many other factors, but without love imbedded in these motivations, they are not as fulfilling as they could be. Many people spend a lifetime wondering why they are unfulfilled. They have money, shelter, and food but cannot seem to realize why they are still unhappy. Love is the key in these situations. Without love, our efforts are fruitless.

Blockages

Blockages in the heart chakra can manifest in many ways, including tension in the area near the location of the chakra. These physical manifestations can occur in the upper back, chest, or ribcage. Shoulders tend to be tight and tense when the heart chakra is unbalanced.

When the heart chakra is blocked, there is difficulty finding love anywhere in life. This means no self-love, no love for others and not love of hobbies or other activities. This is a terrible feeling not to be able to share love or appreciate our surroundings. Depression, self-hatred, and cruel behaviors towards others may be manifestations of a blocked heart chakra.

Without love in our lives there is very little to enjoy. Mundane tasks meant to ensure survival are not fun as they are, let alone if you cannot appreciate them. It may seem simple to find love for many people, but there are just as many who have trouble experiencing this joy. The lack of compassion and care towards other humans and the world is not a desirable life, but learning to open the heart chakra can help immensely with this problem.

Balancing

To balance the heart chakra we need to connect with ourselves on a personal level and try to rebuild our relationship with love. Learning to love oneself is crucial to sharing love with others. Deep breathing and contemplation are great exercises for the heart chakra. In addition, rearranging or cleaning our homes can help start anew in a sense when it comes to self-care. Changing diet and overall aiming to be healthier, goes a long way to help with our perception of ourselves.

This chakra is one of the more complex ones since love is such a mysterious and powerful thing this chakra has a heavy burden to bear. Take great care when working with this chakra, and always try to be compassionate to others, especially the less fortunate.

Attributes

The color of the heart chakra is green. You can wear green or decorate your home in green to help balance this chakra.

The stone attributed to the heart chakra is sapphire. Carry one of these stones or wear it in jewelry. A necklace is best since it will hang near your heart chakra.

The metal of the heart chakra is copper. Wear this metal in jewelry or carry a piece to help balance the chakra.

The mineral of this chakra is potassium. If your heart chakra is unbalanced, you may be ingesting too much or too little of this mineral.

The musical key for this chakra is F. Listen to songs in this key or meditate on the F note to balance the heart chakra.

The seed sound for this chakra is Yam. Chant this sound or listen to recordings of it while meditating to balance the heart chakra.

The thymus gland is associated with the heart chakra. This gland may not function properly if our heart chakra is unbalanced.

The flavors associated with this chakra are astringent in nature. Having too much or too little of these flavors may cause your heart chakra to become unbalanced.

Chapter 9: The Throat Chakra

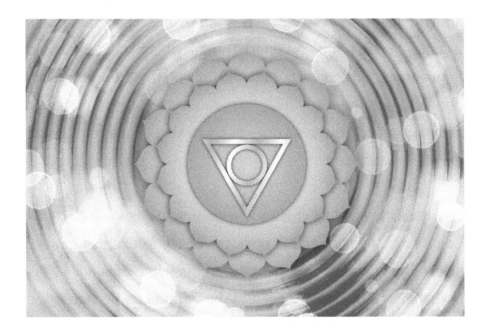

The fifth chakra is know as *Vishuddha*, which translates to "especially pure". The throat chakra is key to communicating and putting our plans into action, in essence it gives voice to our personal truths. We are not able to use language and action to set our plan into motion, then no one will ever hear our dreams. With a foundation of survival instincts, creative inspiration, a sunny battery, and pure love, we can build a balanced life.

Vishuddha

The throat chakra is located at the base of the throat or neck area in the physical body. This chakra is associated with akasha, the element of aether. The throat chakra is attributed to governing our capacity to communicate, both truthfully with our self and honestly with others. If there are problems communicating with loved ones or coworkers your throat chakra may be unbalanced.

The balancing of this chakra is essential for experiencing joy. Socializing, singing, and overall, the ability to express oneself is key to this chakra. For this reason, as you can imagine, the throat chakra is closely linked to the sacral one. If blocked, it could make it problematic for one to experience joy through community and other fun activities.

The throat chakra's image is a sixteen-petaled lotus with a triangle pointing downward and a circle in the center. Being truthful with yourself is key to balancing this chakra. Before you can reach the third eye chakra and experience intuitive and inspirational insight, you must be honest with yourself and work through any personal problems that have lead you to be untruthful and lie to others as well as to yourself.

Honest communication is crucial to developing lifelong relationships and a balanced life. We need to be able to communicate not only with others but also with ourselves sincerely. This communication will allow us to make informed decisions to build upon a firm foundation. If we are not honest with ourselves first, we will not be able to do it with others. Honesty is formed out of love, and we should not be dishonest to our loved ones, nor should we be dishonest towards ourselves. The truth is valued overall throughout life. There is nothing more valuable than the truth. Without truth, there is only chaos and deception.

The throat chakra will be unbalanced if we cannot be truthful with ourselves. Its unbalance manifests in the physical world as fear of public speaking, not being understood, or even struggling to have people listening to you in the first place. The throat chakra governs activities like socializing, negotiations, expression, and in general, any means of communication. Without proper means of communication, the only results are misunderstandings and broken lines of expression.

Blockages

Our throat chakra can manifest ailments when it is blocked near or around the area it resides in. You may have sore throats often, a sore neck or feel sore in the upper spine area of your body. Problems with the mouth or jaw are also common when there are throat chakra blockages.

One of the most prominent side effects of an unbalanced throat chakra is the inability to use language and communication effectively. This can result in overactive talking or interruptive speaking, as well as the inability to speak up when needed. Some may find that they speak and simply aren't heard. Arguments and misunderstanding may ensue as a result of these blockages.

Without effective communication, it is impossible to truly convey our feelings for others. Without proper communication skills, we also cannot contribute positively to society through art, community activities, or industrial progress. We also need to consider that when we say communication we are not only referring to speaking, but also trying to communicate in other ways such as gestures or acts of kindness. These actions may be unsuccessful or interpreted in the wrong ways.

Balancing

To balance the throat chakra, we need to actively engage with our communication skills. Singing, chanting, and openly practicing your public speaking are great exercises to stimulate this chakra. Drinking soothing teas like chamomile or lemon will also help.

You will know when your throat chakra is balanced, as you will be able to speak clearly, truthfully and kindly. It will feel like you know the exact words to speak in each situation, and your words will be helpful, enlightening and able to inspire others.

Practicing the art of silence is also effective for balancing the throat chakra. Sitting quietly in meditation or choosing a whole day to challenge yourself not to speak can be great ways to learn about your impulses and control your urges to interrupt.

Sometimes is just a matter of being mindful and thinking before we speak. If not from me, take it from Buddha: "If you propose to speak always ask yourself, is it true, is it necessary, is it kind."

Attributes

The color of the throat chakra is blue. Wearing this color or decorating your home with this color can help balance the chakra. Perhaps try wearing a blue scarf as well.

The stone associated with the throat chakra is quartz. Carrying this stone or wearing it in jewelry helps to open and balance this chakra. A necklace would be fitting since this chakra is located at the neck.

The metal of this chakra is mercury. Mercury can be used for chakra workings, but this not recommended for beginners since it is highly toxic.

The mineral associated with this chakra is silicon. If your diet is too high or too low in silicon, then your throat chakra may become unbalanced.

The musical key associated with the throat chakra is G. Listening to songs in this key or meditating on the G note will help balance this chakra.

The seed sound associated with this chakra is Ham. Chant this sound or meditate on recordings of this chant to open and balance the throat chakra.

The thyroid gland is associated with this chakra. If your thyroid is not functioning properly, you may have a blocked throat chakra.

The flavor associated with the throat chakra is sour. If you ingest too many sour foods or you do not ingest a sufficient amount of them, can impact the balance of this chakra.

Chapter 10: The Third Eye Chakra

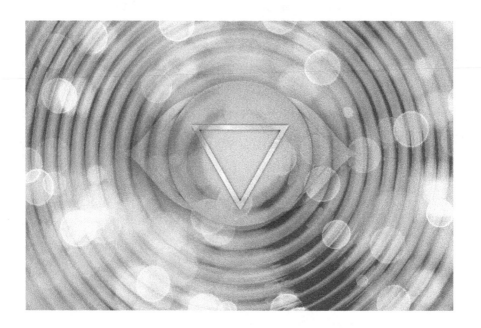

The sixth primary chakra according to Hindu tradition is called *Ajna*, which translates to "authority" or "command". Also known as the "guru chakra" or The third eye chakra mainly deals with intuitive faculties. These faculties can be used to help navigate day to day life in the physical, and also for spiritual progress. The third eye is thought to offer insight into the mysteries of life, while also registering information beyond the surface level and giving insight into our mundane life as well. It is considered to be the seat of the mind, of conscious and unconscious awareness

Ajna

The third eye chakra is known to relate to our pineal gland. Many traditions believe that this gland is responsible for intuitive and spiritual insight. This third eye is located between the eyebrows, just as the pineal gland is located in the same region, but inside of your skull. This chakra is thought to be where the kundalini energy breaks free to offer spiritual awareness and intuitive insight to prepare one for true enlightenment.

We see the third eye symbolically represented in many cultures from around the world. Consider the Egyptian priests with a cobra protruding out of their headdress right where the third eye is located. This can be compared to the serpent kundalini energy as it breaks through the third eye.

The third eye chakra's image is a two-petaled lotus flower with a triangle pointing downward at its center. It is thought that the Nadis cross at this point unifying the female and male channels of energy at the third eye. This breakthrough of the pineal gland is said to destroy duality for the student, allowing them to see the oneness of all things; female and male, light and dark. The student will finally recognize how these forces work together to create a whole universe of existence.

The concept that we can intuitively navigate through our lives is a notion found in many cultures. Consider anytime you've experienced precognition, for example feeling when someone is about to call you, or dreaming of the future. This is the third eye at work, and when balanced, it can access the deepest mysteries and truths of our existence. These skills are challenging to develop, but when we access these powers, we are gifted the most truthful insights about human existence.

Most religions have stories of precognitions and spiritual insight experienced by adherents. These stories can easily be linked to the powers of the third eye chakra. The work we can do with this chakra will allow us to see the truths behind certain events in our life. We will then be able to balance positive and negative forces at work during any given scenario. Being able to have this sight into the truth of reality is a skill that is invaluable for navigating our lives and learning about ourselves as individuals.

Blockages

When the third eye chakra is blocked, it can manifest headaches and migraines that are reoccurring. You may experience lightheadedness, dizziness, or in some cases, even loss of balance.

Since this chakra is closely associated with our intuitive faculties, its blockage can cause us to lose our intuition all together. Lack of insight and inspiration also come along with this chakra's unbalance. Many find that they have no imagination and no sense of wonder or curiosity when this chakra is blocked.

If this chakra is overstimulated people may experience an overactive imagination, leading to hallucinations or intense paranoia. In extreme cases, this may cause insanity or other mental problems, leading to delusion and lack of self-awareness.

Balancing

To balance this chakra, we need to engage our intuitive faculties. We can do this through meditation and visualization, and actively using the imagination. Reading fiction books or keeping a dream journal also do wonders for our intuition.

Taking the time to abandon our agenda and just 'go with the flow' can be very therapeutic for the third eye as well. A spontaneous vacation to someplace away from civilization is recommended.

Attributes

The color associated with the third eye chakra is violet. Wear this color or decorate your home with this color to help balance this chakra.

The stone of the third eye chakra is opal. Carry this stone or wear it in jewelry to help balance this chakra.

The metal of this chakra is silver. Wear jewelry that is made of silver to help stimulate and balance the third eye chakra.

The mineral associated with the third eye chakra is chlorine. If you have too little to too much chlorine in your diet, your third eye chakra may become blocked or unbalanced.

The musical key of this chakra is A. Listening to songs in this key or meditating on the note A will help to balance this chakra.

The seed sound of this chakra is Om. Chant this sound or listen to recordings of these chants to balance the third eye chakra.

The pituitary gland is associated with the third eye chakra. If this gland is not functioning properly, then this chakra may be unbalanced.

The flavor that is associated with this gland is sweetness. If your diet is too sweet or lacks sweetness, your third eye chakra can become unbalanced.

Chapter 11: The Crown Chakra

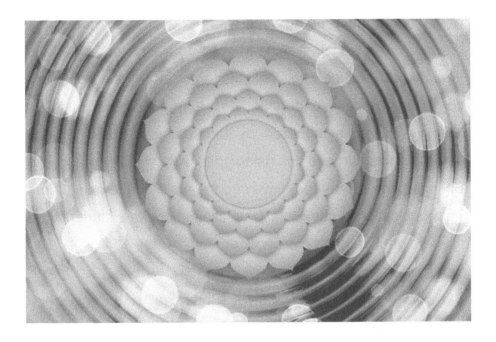

The seventh chakra form the base is the crown chakra is known as *Sahasrara*, which translates to "thousand petaled". It is located at the top of the head or slightly above the head. This chakra is the link between our energetic and physical bodies as well as the forces that are greater than us. Access to the heavens, gods, and goddesses are found through work with the crown chakra.

Sahasrara

The crown chakra is the highest chakra. The ultimate goal of working with these energy centers is to access and open the crown chakra. Accomplishing in opening the crowns chakra is thought to induce an enlightened state, one of pure consciousness and understanding. It is pure consciousness energy. This is symbolized by the feminine Shakti energy completing its purpose and rising up to unite with the masculine Shiva energy. Once again, we see the male and female union. This unification achieves self-realization for the student, the ultimate goal of these chakra workings.

Sahasrara is said to be the most subtle chakra in the system, and it is somewhat hard to explain. Think of it like magnetism. When you hold a magnet to a metal you feel the attraction and tension, you know the magnetism is there, but you do not see that force. Consciousness energy works in a very similar manner, it is everywhere and in everything, connecting us to the entire universe.

Achieving this unification is easier for some people than for others. Once again, practice and experience play a crucial role. Opening this chakra is one of the hardest goals to achieve. Many people have claimed to have experienced such awakening, but in reality, there are more frauds than actual gurus. As a practical guideline, it is safe to say that anyone claiming to be enlightened most certainly is not!

The crown chakra is often referred to as a thousand petaled lotus. With one thousand petals, arranged in 20 layers, each layer with approximately 50 petals, an infinite and almost formless visual that captures the truth of bliss and enlightenment. Reaching this state is similar to the fourth noble truth in Buddhism, the attainment of opening this chakra and enlightenment being one and the same.

The crown chakra is the key to linking our earthly existence to the greater forces of the universe. However, you look at this greater force, whether you refer to it as God or any other name, this force connects with us through the crown chakra.

All spiritual evolution is worked on through the crown chakra. In eastern and Buddhist models to access and open the crown chakra is to reach an enlightened state. This is the ultimate goal of spiritual development and chakra work. Being able to attain this state will take dedication and hard work. Many students will never reach this ultimate goal, but nonetheless, their journeys are fruitful.

We need to stress the point that seeking to reach this state of enlightenment is often a troubling challenge for many students. It is not uncommon for some to become distracted and aggravated when they do not reach an enlightened state. This behavior is contradicting and detrimental to the hard work they may have put into their practice. We need to keep in mind that our journey is the most important, rather than a potential destination.

The crown chakra is not reached unless all other chakras are balanced and open. The Kundalini energy that is dormant at the base of your spine can awaken and led up your spine, climbing the chakras all the way up to the crown chakra. This opening of the crown chakra is often a very intense experience, it may be abrupt, or even gradual over time, but you will certainly know it is happening.

Blockages

Having the crown chakra unbalanced can cause similar physical problems as the third eye chakra. Headaches, brain fog, and lack of intuitive faculties may be related to the crown chakra. If you are close-minded or feel that there is nothing greater than yourself, then you may be experiencing blockages of this chakra.

Since this chakra is related to spiritual endeavor and reaching an enlightened state, its blockage may result in narcissism or extreme self-indulgence in the way a person perceives the world around them. These close-minded ideas are just that, close-minded, you should try to avoid indulging them. If our crown chakra is open, our being is presented before the universe, ready to accept its beauty and vastness. People with a closed mind, do not even consider these experiences to be possible.

While accessing the crown chakra takes a lot of time and effort, its gifts are invaluable. The blocked crown chakra does not see passed material wealth, judging all things on their monetary value. There is no wonder or sense of a greater cause. This chakra is one of the most detrimental when blocked.

Balancing

To balance the crown chakra, we need to see passed our tiny personal world. Mediation, volunteering, and travel are all activities which help to combat a closed mind. Intentionally going outside of your comfort zone, enlarge your horizons, will also help stimulate this chakra.

Religious study and spiritual contemplation go a long way to open this chakra, and it does not have to be any particular religion. The pure contemplation of these grand concepts is enough to help open the crown chakra. Taking time to be grateful and appreciate your life is also a recommended practice.

Attributes

The color associated with the crown chakra is indigo/purple or colorless. Wearing indigo will help to balance this chakra. Additionally, even being nude has proven to help.

The stone associated with the crown chakra is diamond. Wearing this stone in jewelry will help to balance this chakra.

The metal associated with this chakra is gold. Wearing this metal in jewelry will help to open and balance the crown chakra.

The mineral associated with this chakra is fluorine. If your diet is lacking fluorine or too high in fluorine, the crown chakra may become unbalanced.

The musical key associated with the crown chakra is B. Listening to songs in this key or meditating on the B note will help balance this chakra.

The seed sound for this chakra is Om. Chant this sound or listen to recordings of these chants to balance the crown chakra.

The pineal gland is associated with the crown chakra. If your pineal gland does not function properly, then you may have a blocked crown chakra.

There is no flavor associated with the crown chakra.

Conclusion

Thank you for buying and reading Chakras for Beginners. I hope you found it informative and useful, providing you with the foundation and tools you need to start your path and achieve all your goals, whatever they are.

Don't forget that this book is just the beginning. The next step is for you to learn how to practice the concepts you have read about so far. You have moved the first steps in this new path. You will soon find out that the beginning isn't the easiest part.

As we know, the seven-chakra system has seen a long journey making its way west, absorbing new concepts and evolving into the system we know today. As you begin to work with this system, you are taking the first essential steps toward a new life and perspective on the world. Being able to use these skills to improve our lives is not only a cherished gift, but a powerful resource to ensure a fulfilling existence. These secrets of the world are becoming more and more available as the internet connects the world, soon these ideas will be at the core of everyday life, offering insight into the true nature of reality.

Should you wish to learn more and process further down this new path you discovered, please check out my other books on the topic.